St. John's Wort

C.M. Hawken

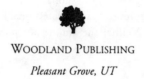

Woodland Publishing

Pleasant Grove, UT

CONTENTS

St. John's Wort

(*Hypericum perforatum*)

Overview

St. John's wort (*Hypericum perforatum*) belongs to the family Hypericaceae, which consists of eight genuses and about 350 species. St. John's wort is a plant whose leaves are whorled, gland-dotted, simple, and usually smooth-margined. Its flowers are five-petalled and yellow with many stamens, which are often united in bundles.

St. John's wort was first known to be used in the Crusades to treat battle wounds. Contemporary research supports this, with various diseases proving Hypericum's worth in aiding all types of topical wounds in their healing and recovery. It is specifically used for putrid leg ulcers that are difficult to heal, and is used to treat many varying septic wounds, boils, and inflammation in cellulite and lymphangitis.[1]

For centuries, St. John's wort has been used to treat disorders of "mood and temperament." Modern research is also backing this up, with several very recent studies demonstrating St. John's wort's ability to treat mild and moderate forms of depression as well and with fewer side effects as the standard antidepressant drugs used.

Recent investigation is also revealing St. John's wort to be helpful for a number of other disorders. Among them is AIDS/HIV, a disease that leads several age/gender groups in cause of death. But St. John's wort is being researched for its ability to hinder viral growth and production, perhaps making it key to at least treating the virus, if not able to cure the disease. *Hypericum* is being used for treatment research of several other virus-caused diseases as well.

Another area in which St. John's wort is showing great promise is that of cancer. Various forms of cancers and growths have been successfully treated with therapies including *Hypericum* or hypericin (one of its compounds). And the list goes on and on. St. John's wort is certainly an herb worth investigating for its seeming abilities to combat various disorders prevalent among us.

Hypericin

One of the reasons St. John's wort is attracting so much interest is because of one of its compounds, hypericin. The journal *Photochemistry-Photobiology* recently published a review of hypericins and the structurally related hypocrellins, giving a favorable outline of the various recent breakthroughs in medicine using these two compounds. The review states,

Hypocrellins and hypericins, structurally related plant pigments isolated from Hypocrella bambuase and Hypericum respectively, are known photodynamic agents. This review summarizes certain significant advances in the phtotophysics, photochemistry and photobiology of these pigments in the last two years and discusses their prospects as novel therapeutic and diagnostic agents in the future . . . In particular, substantial progress has been made in both anticancer and antiviral applications (especially anti-human immunodeficiency virus). . . . The biomedical advances of hypocrellins and hypericins have been further promoted by significant progress in their chemical synthesis and the recent commercialization of . . . hypericins.[2]

The compound hypericin was isolated from St. John's wort in 1942 and has been used as an antidepressant and mood stabilizer for emotionally and mentally disturbed people. Among its many beneficial qualities is that of increasing blood flow to stressed tissue, thereby having a tranquilizing effect. It also reduces the fragility of capillaries and enhances uterine muscle tone because of its ability to increase blood flow.[3] It is this compound that is being extensively researched for its possible therapeutic properties for a variety of diseases, mainly depression, AIDS and other viruses, cancer and sleep disorders.

Extensive research has been done, especially recently, to determine exactly how hypericin works in treating these and other disorders. Nearly all the researchers are saying the same thing—that *Hypericum* (and specifically hypericin) promises significant value to the medical world in overcoming these serious disorders. The following sections discuss the various disorders that are being researched in conjunction with *Hypericum/* hypericin therapy.

Hypericin's Photodynamic Ability

One of hypericin's qualities that enhances its ability to act therapeutically is that of being photodynamic; that is, its different qualities are either initiated by the presence of light or enhanced by it. Most of the contemporary studies dealing with hypericin have in some way or another dealt with how hypericin performs in its various functions when exposed to light. A 1995 study published in *Photochemistry-Photobiology* touts hypericin's therapeutic actions in the viral and cancer worlds, especially when exposed to light. A 1994 *Laryngyscope* study suggested that hypericin has shown the ability to be an effective photosensitizer for certain forms of human cancer. And a 1994 *Photochemistry-Photobiology* study states that "the photocytocidal activity of this quinone on neoplastic cells is superior to that of anti-tumor anthraquinone drugs, such as daunomycin and mitoxanthrone . . ."[4]

The list goes on and on. The consensus seems to be that not only does hypericin possess various therapeutic properties, but that these properties are usually augmented by the presence of light.

THERAPEUTIC APPLICATIONS OF ST. JOHN'S WORT

DEPRESSION—AN OVERVIEW

Depression is a disorder that affects millions of people, both Americans and worldwide. It takes many forms, but is usually marked by sadness, inactivity and heightened self-depreciation. Hopelessness and pessimism are often common symptoms, as are lowered self-esteem, reduced energy and vitality, and loss of the overall capability to enjoy one's existence. Depression is probably the most common psychiatric complaint offered to doctors, and has been described by physicians from at least the time of Hippocrates, who called it "melancholia." The course the disorder runs varies widely from person to person. Depression may be short-term, or may occur repeatedly at short intervals. It may be somewhat permanent, mild or sever, acute or chronic. And who does depression most affect? Rates of incidence are higher among women than men (for varying reasons, some not totally understood). And men are more at risk of suffering from depression as they age, while a woman's peak age for experiencing depression is usually between the ages of 35-45.

Depression is caused by many things—it could come about because of childhood traumas, or because of stressful life events—but more and more, doctors and scientists are pointing to biochemical processes as a main culprit in the onset of depression. Defective regulation of the release of one or more naturally occurring monoamines in the brain—particularly norepinephrine—leads to reduced quantities or reduced activity of these chemicals in the brain, bringing on the depressed mood for most sufferers.

Accompanying the increase in depression cases and the emerging knowledge of its causes has been the rise of drug and other therapies in treating the disorder. The two most important are drug therapy and psychotherapy.

Psychotherapy aims to resolve any underlying psychic conflicts that may be causing the depressed state, while giving emotional support to the patient. This usually involves seeing a psychiatrist and/or psychologist at regular intervals. This also may be accompanied by participation in support groups.

Antidepressant drugs, on the other hand, directly affect the chemistry of the brain and its chemicals, such as the monoamines that are thought to have the most effect on depressed emotional states and moods. The tricyclic antidepressant drugs are thought to work by inhibiting the body's physiological inactivation of the monoamine transmitters. This results in the buildup or accumulation of these neurotransmitters in the brain and allows them to remain in contact with nerve cell receptors longer, thus aiding in elevating the mood of the patient. There are other drugs, called oxidase inhibitors, which interfere with the activity of monoamine oxidase, an enzyme known to be involved in the breakdown of norepinephrine and serotonin.[5]

While drug therapy is something more favorable than continuing suffering from depression, for many persons who take these medications it brings on very undesirable side effects. Uncomfortable physical side effects are among the biggest complaints. Many drug users suffer from sensations of nausea, bloating, indigestion, abdominal cramping and diarrhea, and other gastrointestinal discomforts. Dizziness is often a common complaint, and there are many others.

For decades, St. John's wort has been utilized as a mood elevator, antidepressant and overall mental stimulant. As mentioned before, since times as far back as the Crusades do we have record of St. John's wort being used in this and other capacities. Wounds were treated with the herb's extracted oil, the insane were given the herb for its effect on both the nervous system and brain, and it was even used to cast out evil spirits (which often is linked to hallucinations and other mental instability).

More recent uses in "folk" or nonstandard medicine point to St. John's wort's effective use not only as an antidepressant and nervous system tonic, but also for neuralgia, wounds, kidney problems, its anti-inflammatory and antibacterial properties, and of very recent interest, its use as an AIDS virus inhibitor. Michael Murray, in his book *Natural Alternatives to Over-the-Counter Drugs,* points to St. John's wort's uses for the previously listed uses, and the results of several recent clinical studies. Rebecca Flynn and Mark Roest also outline very well the benefits of the herb as shown in medical and other tests.[6] The information coming from both the folk medicine and the clinical medicine worlds indicates that St. John's wort possesses effective and safe healing properties for several disorders and ailments, and potentially many more.

DEPRESSION—STANDARD AND ALTERNATIVE TREATMENTS

Depression is a commonly occurring disorder; according to one recently published report, it affects nearly 17 percent of all Americans for the length of their lives.[7] Because depression often involves a complex mixture of severity, length, and mode of treatment, it is often a difficult decision for doctors and patients alike to decide how to treat the depression. Many practitioners and patients are reluctant to use antidepressant drugs because of associated side effects. It seems logical, then that any additional forms of treatment with little risk, credible benefit, and moderate cost would be a useful addition to depression management.

Extracts of St. John's wort have long been used in "folk" medicine for a range of symptoms and problems, including mood and depression disorders. Extracts of St. John's wort are licensed in Germany for the treatment of "anxiety and depressive and sleep disorders." In 1993, more than 2.7 million prescriptions of *Hypericum* were counted in the seven most popular preparations in Germany.[8] In the past ten years, several randomized clinical trials have compared the effects of pharmaceutical preparations of *Hypericum* with placebo and common antidepressants, with nearly all showing favorable practical application of *Hypericum* treatments for depression and other related disorders.

RECENT RESEARCH

A recent study (August, 1996) exploring the effect of *Hypericum perforatum* on depression revealed some fairly stunning results. The *British Medical Journal* published the results of one major studies, which consisted of twenty-three randomized trials, including a total of 1757 outpatients with mainly mild or moderately severe depressive disorders. Testing was conducted with single preparations and combinations of extracts of the plant, and with placebo and anther drug treatment.

As just mentioned, the results were very promising. In all aspects of the study, *Hypericum* extracts were shown to be "significantly superior" to placebo and similarly effective as standard antidepressants. There were nearly twice the number, percentage-wise, of dropouts due to side effects from the standard drugs than those taking the *Hypericum* extracts. Side effects occurred in eighty-four patients using standard antidepressants, while only fifty patients taking the *Hypericum* extracts experienced side effects. And the scores on the Hamilton depression scale, which measures severity of one's depression, showed those taking *Hypericum* treatments scored slightly higher than those taking the standard antidepressant and significantly higher than those taking the placebo.[9] This study provides some firm ground for St. John's wort to stand on in the treatment of depression, both in sheer numbers and its quality of treatment.

Another contemporary study, carried out in 1995 by Witte, et. al, showed the Linde study to be accurate in its findings. This particular study, carried out as a multicenter, placebo-controlled double-blind trial, used a highly concentrated *Hypericum* preparation to treat ninety-seven outpatients. The course of the illness was assessed with the Hamilton Depression Scale, the von Zerssen Depressivity Scale and the Clinical Global Impression Scale. The authors of the study noted this in their abstract:

> Treatment resulted in an appreciable improvement in the symptoms of depression, and the seventy percent response rate (n=43) corresponded to that of chemical antidepressants. The preparation also showed an anxiolytic effect. The substance [hypericum] was extremely well tolerated, and no side effects were reported by any of the patients.[10]

Again, this study's findings correlate that of the Linde and other studies in that treatment with *Hypericum* is at least as effective as standard synthetic antidepressants without producing near the number of side effects.

The *Nursing Times* also reported on recent findings dealing with *Hypericum's* effect on depression. Stating that psychiatric medications are notorious for their undesirable side effects, and that the need for safer antidepressants is widely acknowledged, the blurb refers to a double-blind study, done by G. Harrer and H. Sommer (published in *Phytomedicine*, 1994 (1): 3-8), using St. John's wort on 105 patients experiencing mild to moderate depression. They were aged twenty to sixty-four and had diagnoses of "neurotic depression or temporary depressive mood." Patients were divided into two groups and monitored over four weeks, with one group receiving 300 mg of *Hypericum* extract three times daily and the other group receiving a placebo. All patients received psychiatric evaluations before the start of the study and after two and four weeks of treatment.[11]

The results of the study support the findings of other recent studies dealing with *Hypericum* and depression: 67 percent of the *Hypericum* group had responded positively to the treatment without any adverse side effects, whereas only 28 percent of the placebo group displayed any improvement. Harrer and Sommer state that the patients treated were experiencing strictly mild forms of depression; combining this with the study's results and the results of other studies suggest that *Hypericum* treatment can be a very effective treatment for mild to moderate depression without severe side effects. The authors themselves even recommended that *Hypericum* should be considered as a remedy of choice. [12]

These and other studies point to the strong possibility of using St. John's wort, and specifically hypericin, on a wide scale to treat various forms of depression.

Linde's study suggests that St. John's wort may have its most valuable asset in that of few or no side effects, something many sufferers of depression are very concerned about. The authors do note, however, that more research is necessary, especially in determining the severity and nature of depression, length of treatment, treatment dosage, preparation of *Hypericum* extracts, and occurrence of long-term side effects. Nevertheless, the results of this study and others are extremely promising for the millions of those who suffer from depression.

Alcohol and Depression

Depression is often a result of other disorders. A recent study conducted by the Ukranian team of A. Krylov, et. al, treated fifty-seven outpatients with alcoholism and accompanying diseases of the digestive organs (such as peptic ulcers and chronic gastritis). The duration of the treatment lasted two months, with one-glass treatments occurring four to five times daily. The study proved St. John's wort effective (when combined with rational psychotherapy) in treating the alcoholism-related depression and also in treating the gastrointestinal disorders.[13]

ANTIVIRAL PROPERTIES

As stated previously, hypericin has recently gained much of the medical world's respect as an antiviral agent, with activity against a broad range of enveloped viruses and retroviruses. The effective virucidal activity emanates from a combination of photodynamic and lipophilic properties. A recent article in the journal *Transfusion* details exactly how hypericin works in inhibiting viral activity among cells:

> Hypericin binds cell membranes (and, by inference, virus membranes) and crosslinks virus capsid proteins. This action results in a loss of infectivity and an inability to retrieve the reverse transcriptase enzymatic activity from the virion.[14]

Another recent study, carried out in 1991, focused on hypericin's ability to inhibit virus activity, more specifically, in the murine cytomegalovirus (MCMV), Sindbis virus, and human immunodeficiency virus type 1 (HIV-1). The Sindbis virus was significantly more sensitive than the MCMV virus. The inactivated MCMV, when used to infect cells, was incapable of synthesizing early or late viral antigens. In addition to the direct virucidal effect, when hypericin was added to cells infected with viable MCMV, inhibition was also observed, particularly when the compound was added in the first two hours of infection. The researchers also indicated that the effect was aided significantly by visible light, pointing again to the plant's photodynamic property.

The study states that hypericin appears to have two modes of antiviral activity: ". . . one directed at the virions, possibly on membrane components, and the other directed at virus-infected cells. Both activities are substantially enhanced by light."[15] And there are other viruses that fall under St. John's wort's antiviral blanket. Contemporary research points to the equine infectious anemia virus, the lentivirus, the Sindbid virus, the radiation leukemia virus, and most importantly, the human immunodeficiency virus (HIV).

St. John's Wort and AIDS/HIV

In 1991, some of the first work focusing on St. John's wort's effects on AIDS and the HIV virus began. *Science* magazine reported on the first study using the isolated hypericin, a key compound in *Hypericum*.[16] Fred Valentine and Howard Hochster, researchers at New York University Medical Center, began one of the first studies looking at how hypericin can help uninfected T-cells from being infected with the AIDS virus in a cell culture. Their focus was on hypericin because it is a virucidal agent, meaning it can precisely target new virus particles and prevent them from infecting other cells.

The only two drugs at that time approved for treating HIV infection—AZT and ddI—work by interfering with the key viral enzyme, reverse transcriptase. Since hypericin works more effectively than many drugs in regards to the reverse transcriptase phase, and since many animal tests have shown that it has low toxicity at therapeutic doses, researchers (including Valentine and Hochster) began these studies largely hoping that not only would hypericin work on its own, but that it would have a sort of synergistic effect when used with either AZT or ddI. [17]

Additional studies are pointing to St. John's wort, and more so, hypericin, as having great potential in treating HIV. Acosta and Fletcher recently detailed the processes in which the human immunodeficiency virus works to infect human cells, and point out that hypericin is at least somewhat effective in inhibiting the four main phases of virus "growth"—binding and entry, reverse transcriptase, transcription and translation, and viral maturation and budding (the researchers note that hypericin is especially effective in binding and entry, the first phase.) This denotes that hypericin could eventually have special importance in completely stifling the development of the growth of any virus, and most importantly, that of the HIV virus.[18]

Another study assessing the use and attitudes of HIV sufferers concerning the use of more alternative treatments for the virus as opposed to clinical drug therapies showed both an extensive use of unconventional therapies and a very favorable response to using the alternative treatments, which, of course, St. John's wort was among. "Participants at all sites expressed positive views upon increasing unconventional remedies."[19] The fact is that the world of synthetic medicines has been basically ineffective in not only treating and relieving the symptoms of AIDS, but also in finding a cure for the dreaded disease. Sufferers are giving alternative therapies a try, and the results are very promising.

A 1995 review appearing in *Photochemisty-Photobiology* treated the photodynamic properties of both hypericin and the structurally related hypocrellins for their anticancer and antiviral properties (especially the anti-human immunodeficiency virus). This article states that the

promising anticancer and antiviral results obtained both in vitro and in vivo [in differing studies] have led to intensive investigation into their photo-physical and photo-chemical processes, especially kinetic studies of their intramolecular proton transfer . . . The biomedical advances of hypericins have been further promoted by significant progress in their chemical synthesis and the recent commercialization of . . . hypericin.[20]

Another study published in the September 1994 issue of *Photochemistry-Photobiology* gave hypericin the upper hand over the hypocrellins in treating HIV. Just one more vote in favor of promoting the use of St. John's wort, and more specifically, hypericin, for use in treating HIV and in overall clinical medicine.

SLEEP DISORDERS

Among the many ailments that often accompany middle and old age are various sleep disorders: insomnia, intermittent waking, sleep duration, and an overall poor sleep quality. The medical world has produced numerous synthetic drugs to deal with these disorders; however, most aren't completely effective and produce undesirable side effects as well. Recent research suggests that St. John's wort may be able to improve one's sleep, especially that of older persons. A 1994 double-blind, placebo-controlled study published in the *Journal of Geriatric Psychiatry and Neurology* showed that *Hypericum* extracts gave the benefit of increased deep sleep during the total sleeping period of the patients. It explains,

A hypostatic influence of the REM sleep phases, which is typical for tricyclic antidepressants and MAO inhibitors, could not be shown for this phytopharmacon [*Hypericum*]. Instead, LI 160 [*Hypericum*] induced an increase of deep sleep during the total sleeping period. This could be shown consistently in the visual analysis of the sleeping phases 3 and 4, as well as in the automatic analysis of slow-wave EEG activities.

The study also makes an interesting connection between sleep and depression; that being many standard antidepressants and MAO inhibitors used to treat people who suffer from depression cause a decrease in deep sleep. As discussed earlier, St. John's wort has shown great promise in treating depressed persons. So, besides helping people with sleep disorders, when used as an antidepressant, it gives antidepressant properties without the side effect of decreased deep sleep.[21] This is certainly another valuable quality St. John's wort has shown to possess.

WOUNDS

St. John's wort oil has long been held in high esteem for treatment of all types of abrasions and wounds. Its fame was reputedly tested time and time again on the battlefields of the Crusades. More modern tests using the oil have proved its reputation. The oil, which does not contain hypericin, contains another valuable compound, hyperforin, which is mainly responsible for the oil's therapeutic properties. Though somewhat difficult to isolate and preserve for extended periods of time, hyperforin has shown considerable promise as a primary component in salves or dressings for topical and other wounds. It only makes sense that in being able to withstand and inhibit bacterial and viral growth, St. John's wort can effectively aid topical wounds in their healing and recovery.

Cancer/Tumors

St. John's wort, and more specifically, hypericin, has an outstanding ability to work favorably at the cell level against normally destructive invaders like viruses and bacterias. But these are not the only destructive agents that are being targeted by researchers in *Hypericum* research. Hypericin has been shown in various recent studies to work very effectively against cancerous cells and tumors of varying kinds.

The April 1996 issue of *Laryngyscope* reported that hypericin is showing great potential in targeting human cancer growths through what is called "phototargeting," a process that uses laser activation of hypericin, along with chemotherapy, for improved results in inhibiting the growth of cancerous cells. The study states,

> These results show that hypericin is a sensitive agent for phototherapy of human cancer cells in vitro and indicate that this drug may be useful for tumor targeting via minimally invasive imaging-guided laser fiber optics.[22]

Another recent study commented on the use of hypericin in treating human cancer cells, saying that "the nucleus of the cell . . . is the target for the toxic action of hypericin." The study pointed out that the compound is well distributed throughout the cells, indicating that its value as an anticancer agent remains high.[23]

Yet another study points to the photodynamic qualities of hypericin in combating cancerous cells. The study's results suggest that hypericin "has considerable potential for use as a sensitizer in the PDT [photodynamic therapy] of cancer." And when hypericin was used in conjunction with other "scavenging" agents, its inhibitory abilities were greatly enhanced.

Again, with such promising results from clinical studies, St. John's wort (and hypericin) is perhaps opening the way to curing one of our most devastating diseases, cancer. Further research could quickly finalize a cure.

BLOOD TRANSFUSIONS

With the increasing rates of several blood-carried diseases (like AIDS), blood transfusion and blood donation rates are declining. Ensuring that donated blood is not "contaminated" by disease dictates that fewer people can donate blood, while fear of being contaminated by blood tainted by blood usually dissuades physicians from requiring blood transfusions unless absolutely necessary. Finding some sort of treatment of tainted blood would not only save money and time, but also calm fears about the possibility of being infected with a potentially serious disease through a blood transfusion. *Hypericum* is showing great promise in being able to treat blood contaminated by viruses. A recent *Transfusion* study states,

> Since hypericin is devoid of adverse action in most blood components and blood analyses, it is investigated as an additive with potential to inactivate infective viruses in blood components intended for transfusion. . . . Complete inactivation of 10 (6) tissue culture-infective doses of human immunodeficiency virus was obtained in whole blood and in diluted packed red cells after illumination with fluorescent light for 1 hour. Loss of viral infectivity to cultured CEM cells has been monitored by use of a detection assay for human immunodeficiency virus p55 in enzyme-linked immunosorbent assay and cytopathic assays. In physiologic media, hypericin interacts with albumin and lipoproteins, retaining the virucidal activity in bound form. . . . The apparent transfusibility of hypericin, taken together with the efficacy of the virucidal activity, the broad range of enveloped viruses affected, and the absence of adverse effects on stored red cells, may render hypericin useful for inactivation of infectious viruses in red cells.[24]

SAFETY

Though research is still ongoing as to the specific actions of St. John's wort and its constituents, it has been established that St. John's wort is quite safe, especially when used as directed. Various studies back up the plant's therapeutic properties and safe use, as well as provide technical information as to what makes St. John's wort function. A 1994 study gives very technical information as to how hypericin works and the optimal methods of extraction, concentration and storage.[25] There have been reports of phototoxicity in animals when taken in extremely large doses, and long-term studies are relatively few in number, but the overall consensus seems to be that *Hypericum* is a safe and effective medicinal herb.

PRIMARY USES

- DEPRESSION
- NERVOUS DISORDERS
- EMOTIONAL/MENTAL REGULATOR
- VIRAL INFECTIONS
- TUMOR AND CANCER RETARDANT
- AIDS VIRUS INHIBITOR
- SEPTIC WOUNDS/ BOILS
- BLOOD TREATMENT

ENDNOTES

1. Ritchason, Jack. *Little Herb Encyclopedia.* (Pleasant Grove, UT: Woodland Publishing, 1994; 208-9).
2. Diwu, Z. "Novel Therapeutic and Diagnostic Applications of Hypocrellins and Hypericins." *Photochemistry-Photobiology,* 1995, 61(6) 529-39.
3. Ritchason, 208.
4. Andreoni, A. et al. "Laser Photosensitization of Cells by Hypericin." *Photochemistry-Photobiology,* 1996, 59(5): 529-33.
5. (Encyclopedia Britannica, 1993: 8, p.21
6. Flynn, Rebecca, M.S. and Roest, Mark. *Your Guide to Standardized Herbal Products.* (Prescott, Az..: One World Press, 1995, 73-4.
7. Linde, et al. "St. John's Wort for Depression — An Overview and Meta-Analysis of Randomised Clinical Trials." *The British Medical Journal.* 1996, 313(7052): 253.
8. Lohse, Mueller et al. *Arzneiverordnungreport '94.* 1994: 354.
9. Linde, et al., 254
10. Witte, et al.
11. Jackson, Adam. "Herbal Help for Depression." *Nursing Times,* 1995: 9(30): 49.
12. Harrer, G.; H. Sommer. "Treatment of Mild/Moderate Depression with *Hypericum.*" *Phytomedicine.* 1994, 1: 3-8.
13. Krylov, A., Ibatov A. "The Use of an Infusion of St. John's Wort in the Combined Treatment of Alcoholics with Peptic Ulcer and Chronic Gastritis." *Vrach.-Delo.* 1993

Feb.-Mar.(2-3): 146-8.

14. Lavie, G. et. al. "Hypericin as an Inactivator of Infectious Viruses in Blood Components." *Transfusion.* 1995, May 35(5): 392-400.

15. Hudson, J.B., Lopez-Bazzocchi, I., Towers, G.H. "Antiviral Activities of Hypericin." *Antiviral—Res.* 1991, Feb. 15(2): 101-12.

16. *Science,* 1991, 254: 522.

17. Ibid.

18. *American Journal of Hospital Pharmacy.* 1994, 51(18): 2251-67.

19. *Journal of Association of Nurses Aids Care.* 1995, Jan-Feb.: 225.

20. Diwu, 34.

21. Schulz, H. "Effects of hypericum extract on the sleep EEG in older volunteers." *The Journal of Geriatry, Psychiatry and Neurology.* 1994, Oct., 7: S39-43.

22. Vander Werf, QM. et al. "Hypericin: a new laser phototargeting agent for human cancer cells." *Lanryngyscope.* 1996, April, 106: 479-83.

23. Miskovsky, P., et al. " Subcellular Distribution of Hypericin in Human Cancer Cells." *Photochem-Photobiol,* 1995, Sept. 62(3): 546-9.

24. "Hypericin as an inactivator of infectious viruses in blood components," *Transfusion,* 1995, May 35(5): 392-400.

25. Wagner, H. and S. Bladt. "Pharmaceutical Quality of *Hypericum* Extracts." *Journal of Geriatry, Psychiatry and Neurology.* Oct. 7, 1994: S65-8.